Introduction

In this book I will share with you a one-month program that can reverse osteoarthritis, rheumatoid arthritis, gouty arthritis, bursitis, fibromyalgia and many of the chronic diseases of aging. I'm not talking about symptom relief only! This comprehensive program, when administered properly, has the power to reverse these conditions permanently!

True health comes from observing the laws of Nature which govern the function and health of the body, mind and spirit. Lately, medicine has been rediscovering that Nature has the answer to most, if not all, of man's health problems. Well, once again, Nature has proven to be far superior in treating the diseases of aging, more so than all of man's medications, by providing us with cetyl myristoleate. This product by itself can increase the quality of your life by 75%–80%. And combined with the synergistic products I will recommend in this book, it can restore your body to almost perfect health.

What Is Arthritis?

Arthritis is inflammation of a joint or joints and the surrounding tissues including tendons, ligaments, and cartilage. Its effects can range from minimal pain, stiffness, and joint swelling to deformity of the joints, crippling and total disability. The three most common types of arthritis are osteoarthritis, rheumatoid arthritis, and gout. By the time we reach 50 years of age, 80% of us will develop osteoarthritis. Presently, one third of the entire adult population suffers with osteoarthritis, often referred to as degenerative joint disease. Almost two and one-half million Americans are afflicted with rheumatoid arthritis—twice as many women as men. Juvenile rheumatoid arthritis affects 71,000 young Americans (aged 18 and under)—six times as many girls as boys. And currently, over one million Americans have been diagnosed with gout, with men being four times more likely than women to develop this painful condition.

What Causes Arthritis?

The causes of arthritis are varied and many. These include trauma with joint instability, aging with increased body weight (causing increased weight-bearing on the joints), altered biochemistry, hormonal changes, and genetic factors. It is now also accepted among most rheumatologists and allergists that some people have allergy-induced arthritis. And mental-emotional stresses induce cortisone deficiencies in the body, which can also be a factor in some forms of arthritis.

Osteoarthritis

Osteoarthritis, also known as degenerative joint disease, is related to the wear and tear of aging and involves deterioration of the cartilage at the ends of the bones. The cartilage then becomes rough and the tendons, muscles, and ligaments holding the joint together become weakened. The body's attempt to stabilize the joint results in the formation of bony spurs or osteophytes. This process

Zoller

Cetyl **CMO** Myristoleate

by Chuck Cochran, D.C., F.C.T.S. - Revised 3rd edition, March, 1997

Published by: Healing Wisdom Publications, 2067 Broadway, New York, NY 10023

About the Author .... **Chuck Cochran, D.C.**

Dr. Cochran comes from a family that has always tried to incorporate attitude, proper nutrition, prevention of disease, and education into healthcare. His stepfather is a chiropractor who, in fact, is still practicing in Sacramento, California, and his mother is a self-taught nutritionist who helped advise patients in her husbands's office for over 30 years.

Dr. Cochran and his brother are graduates of Palmer College in Davenport, Iowa. Since graduation in 1984, his postgraduate education has included programs in skeletal radiography, diagnosis and treatment of soft tissue injuries, operation and diagnostic procedures using thermographic (heat pictures) techniques, and philosophy and clinical techniques of acupuncture.

He has been in private practice since 1984 and during this time owned and operated a multi-disciplinary clinic that included practitioners from four different philosophical backgrounds. He's also had the opportunity to teach college-level human anatomy and physiology and for one year was the chief of operations of a very large nutritional company. Presently, he co-owns Global Nutriceuticals, LLC, a company which specializes in sourcing cutting-edge nutritional products and formulating specialty formulas.

He loves to teach and, consequently, finds himself doing radio shows and speaking to local groups on chiropractic and nutrition. He and his wife, Jeannie, are presently living in Aptos, California.

Disclaimer:
The information in this book is intended for eductational purposes only, and not as a substitute for individual medical attention, or as a specific treatment or a cure for a specific illness. The author and Healing Wisdom Publications shall not be held liable or responsible to any person or entity for any claim of loss, damage, or injury due to the information or inferred recommendations in this book.

TABLE OF CONTENTS

Introduction ii

What Is Arthritis? .... 1.

What Causes Arthritis? .... 1.
- Osteoarthritis .... 1.
- Rheumatoid Arthritis .... 2.
- Gout .... 2.

Now What Is This Stuff, Cetyl Myristoleate? .... 2.

How Was Cetyl Myristoleate Discovered? .... 4.

Adjunctive Nutritional Therapies .... 6.
- Glucosamine .... 7.
- Sea Cucumber Extract .... 8.
- Hydrolyzed Cartilage .... 9.
- Methylsulfonylmethane .... 9.

Clinical Results .... 9.

Some Considerations when Purchasing Cetyl Myristoleate .... 9.

Complementary Treatment and Prevention of Arthritis .... 11.
- Diet and Nutrition .... 12.
- Detoxification .... 14.
  - Colon .... 14.
  - Liver .... 14.
  - Kidneys .... 15.
  - Skin .... 15.
  - Lungs .... 15.

Some Final Thoughts .... 18.

Questions and Answers .... 19.

can be accelerated by being overweight, joint injuries, inadequate diet and improper or no exercise.

Rheumatoid Arthritis

Rheumatoid arthritis is a chronic inflammatory condition that affects the entire body, including the synovial membranes which surround the lubricating fluid (synovial fluid) in the joints. It is an autoimmune disease, a condition in which the body's immune system attacks its own tissues. Rheumatoid arthritis involves multiple joints and not only results in swelling, stiffness, pain and partial dislocation of the joints, but also anemia, fatigue, fever, weight loss and crippling. Causes of this inflammatory reaction include genetic susceptibility, life-style factors, nutritional factors, food allergies and microorganisms. One of the most recent theories is abnormal permeability of the intestinal wall which allows incompletely digested foods to pass through into the blood stream. These large food particles in the blood cause an immune disturbance in which the body's own immune system attacks tissues around the joints.

Gout

Gout is a type of arthritis caused by increased levels of uric acid in the body's fluids. This uric acid helps to form crystals which become deposited in the joints and other tissues, including the kidneys, causing considerable damage that results in inflammation. Gout is often referred to as "the rich man's disease" and historically was associated with affluence. This traditional picture does have basis in reality, as meats, particularly organ meats, cause increased uric acid and alcohol slows down the elimination of uric acid by the kidneys.

Now What Is This Stuff, Cetyl Myristoleate?

I don't want to get too technical in this book, and since most of my readers are not chemists—and this includes the author—I'll try to keep this simple. Cetyl myristoleate is an ester of a fatty acid. This sounds too much like chemistry to me! Let's see if I can start this a little simpler. Fatty acids are the individual components of oils in the same way that amino acids are the building blocks of proteins. Polyunsaturated fatty acids, such as linoleic acid and linolenic acid, are crucial to life and are called essential fatty acids. Monounsaturated oils such as oleic acid can be abundantly found in such oils as olive oil. These are the good oils. Nutritionists now know that daily consumption of the good oils do more to reduce the bad cholesterol (LDL) and increase the good cholesterol (HDL) than cholesterol present in your diet.

Now if we take a fatty acid, myristoleaic acid, and combine it with a long-chain alcohol molecule, cetyl alcohol, we have created an ester of this fatty acid called cetyl myristoleate. Both of these molecules occur in nature. Cetyl alcohol was first derived from the oil of the sperm whale, but now is obtained from palmitic acid (a saturated fatty acid) found in coconut and palm oils. Myristoleaic acid is found in very small percentages in all fats and oils. Historically, many of these products were used in the cosmetic industry because of their ability to act as lubricants. One of the mechanisms of cetyl myristoleate is as a super lubricant (surfactant), a kind of WD-40 for the joints. A surfactant not only has a dissolving or thinning action, it also makes other products easier to absorb.

Concerning the treatment for arthritis, how can one product address all of the causes of this complex disease? Cetyl myristoleate seems to function in three very different capacities. First, as mentioned above it serves as a surfactant and not only lubricates the involved joints, but also lubricates the entire body, making muscles glide more smoothly over other muscles, bursas, and bones and at the same time softens these tissues making them more pliable. Secondly, it functions as an immune system modulator. This is the reason it has been found to be so effective in treating autoimmune diseases such as rheumatoid arthritis, systemic lupus erythematosus, and multiple sclerosis. And last, it functions like a fatty acid in that it mediates inflammatory processes. When cooled, cetyl myristoleate is a waxy substance and, at room temperature, it has a buttery consistency.

How Was Cetyl Myristoleate Discovered?

The discovery of cetyl myristoleate is a fascinating and a disturbing story. It actually begins in 1962 when Dr. Harry W. Diehl, a researcher for the National Institutes for Health, was given an assignment to create arthritis in a certain group of mice to test a drug. An injection of inactive Mycobacterium butyricum, also referred to as Freund's Adjuvant, will induce arthritic symptoms in most animals. So Harry proceeded to inject these Swiss Albino mice with this toxin, and discovered that these little mice did not develop arthritis. As a researcher, I'm sure this peaked his curiosity. What did the Swiss Albino mouse have in its body that prevented it from getting arthritis? Harry Diehl worked on this project for two years, and in 1964, he isolated a substance that was unique to this particular mouse. It turned out to be a fatty acid ester that we now know as cetyl myristoleate.

The next step was to see if this substance could prevent arthritis in other animals. He proceeded to inject the cetyl myristoleate into rats that he knew could develop arthritis and then injected them again with the Freund's Adjuvant. Not only did the rats remain arthritis-free, but they grew an average of 5.7 times as much as the control group that did not receive the cetyl myristoleate injections.

What a discovery! It should have been announced from the highest towers in every city of the world. Instead, nothing was done about this fantastic event until 1976 when Dr. Diehl applied for a use-patent for the purpose of preventing rheumatoid arthritis. Apparently, funding was stopped on his project. Could it be that since no product patent was obtainable (you can't patent a product that occurs naturally), the powers that be halted the research since no money could be made. Whoops! I sound a little cynical.

In 1985, Dr. Diehl finished his own research and determined that it was safe for human use and started sharing cetyl myristoleate with family and friends. In 1991, he developed osteoarthritis in his own hands and feet, and I'm told that he injected himself with one gram of this substance. His arthritis symptoms left, never to return. According to Dr. Diehl, symptom relief occurred 98% of the time with 80% experiencing total relief of symptoms. Some of his earlier volunteers have been arthritis-free for over nine years. In November of 1993 he made his discovery public by publishing his research in The Journal of Pharmaceutical Sciences. According to Dr. Diehl's research, a *minimum* (more is better) of 17 grams of cetyl myristoleate is required to prevent arthritis in an average (175 lb.) individual.

Since that time, healthcare practitioners who use safe, drug-alternative methods have been discovering this wonderful product and have found it to be just as Harry Diehl had said. I have used it myself and now sleep on a arthritic shoulder that I haven't slept on since 1967 when I was involved in a motorcycle accident. I have shared it with hundreds of patients and have found its effectiveness truly amazing. Its true reason for being, that has yet to be explored, however, is in the prevention of inflammatory diseases.

Clinical Results

A multi-center clinical research study involving 431 patients with various forms of arthritis was performed in 1996, using various established measurement criteria including joint swelling joint pain, chest expansion, blood analysis, and patient and doctor assessments. The remarkable results showed significant improvement in 63.3% of those using cetyl myristoleate by itself and 88.6% (patient's assessment and doctor's assessment were within a 4% range) improvement in those given cetyl myristoleate combined with glucosamine, sea cucumber, and hydrolyzed cartilage along with a topical 25% lotion of cetyl myristoleate. In comparison, only 16.6% of the placebo group showed improvement.

If a major drug company released an arthiritis treatment that was only 50% effective, this information would appear in the world media within days!

Adjunctive Nutritional Therapies

However fantastic this product is, its effectiveness can be improved by another 10%–20% by adding a few additional natural ingredients. In nature, we observe that nothing works or stands alone. There is always a collaboration or supporting complimentary action which makes things happen. This interaction, when the total effect is greater than the sum of the individual effects, is called synergism.

I bring this to your attention because I have found many applications of synergism in the formulation of natural remedies for the treating of my patients. If two separate substances help in the same condition, the combination of these substances often produces a total effect far greater than the use of only one of the substances.

In using fatty acid esters, we discovered that results were much longer lasting when we developed a comprehensive program. This treatment protocol not only combines cetyl myristoleate with other complementary or synergistic oils that enhance its performance, but we have included several other time-honored, clinic-tested natural substances that have been found very effective in the treatment of all arthritic conditions.

This includes one product that combines of glucosamine, sea cucumber extract, hydrolyzed cartilage and methylsulfonylmethane in a capsule to be taken two capsules three times daily. And last, a topical cream that contains cetyl myristoleate and a carrier that can be applied over the involved joints. The entire program is designed to be completed in one month. Even though most patients are symptom-free at this point, I recommend the continued use of the support capsules for at least another 3–4 months. In approximately 2% of the population, one more complete program may be necessary, but I recommend waiting 2–3 weeks before starting another session. Occasionally the desired effects may take up to 6 weeks. Several of my patients have experienced a continuing decrease in symptoms even after the one-month recommended treatment is completed.

Glucosamine

Glucosamine has had more of an impact on my life and the lives of all my patients suffering from the various forms of arthritis than any other one product, prior to cetyl myristoleate. Prior to my discovery of glucosamine in 1989, I was forced to have regular steroid injections into my shoulder to relieve the symptoms of traumatic arthritis. On one occasion, it became so painful that in spite of all the therapies I had available to me, I was forced to quit my practice of chiropractic. Fortunately, glucosamine became available about that time and, after three months of daily use, all my shoulder symptoms were gone and I was able to return to work!

Glucosamine is an amino sugar necessary for the construction of connective tissue. It is produced by the body and is an integral part in the production of nails, tendons, skin, eyes, synovial fluid (fluid found in the joints that provides nutrients and lubrication), bone, ligaments, heart valves, and mucous secretions of the digestive, respiratory and urinary tracts. Absence of glucosamine in the diet can result in early aging of cells and loss of cellular function resulting in premature cell death. It has been found when compared to nonsteroidal, antiinflammatory drugs (NSAID) to be far superior in treating osteoarthritis. Remember, NSAIDs are symptom relievers only and actually inhibit cartilage repair!

Glucosamine actually helps to rebuild the damaged cartilage in the joint. This process can take weeks or months to accomplish depending on the extensiveness of joint damage, and consequently, many people have given up on this wonderful product because symptom relief was too slow in coming. Added to cetyl myristoleate, we have an unbeatable combination. This is a product that you should continue to use after the recommended cetyl myristoleate program is completed to ensure that the body is provided with all of the building blocks needed to reconstruct the damaged joint tissues.

Sea Cucumber Extract

The vegetable of the deep, according to one well known health care provider and author, emits defensive toxins that have been found to be powerful anti-inflammatories and useful in the treatment of all arthritic conditions, as well as tendonitis, bursitis, myofascitis, and sports injuries. According to this source, homeopathic dilutions of these toxins are about 25 times more effective than aspirin in reducing inflammation and have a greater lasting effect!

Sea cucumber has been used in Traditional Chinese Medicine (TCM) for hundreds of years, and its medicinal use dates back thousands of years. In a modern study, about 84% of those using it for rheumatoid arthritis had mild to significant objective and subjective improvement.

A sea cucumber product is now registered for over-the-counter sale in Australia and New Zealand as a treatment for arthritis.

Hydrolyzed Cartilage

Cartilage is rich in mucopolysaccharides, large molecules which are found in all our joints, blood vessels, and organs. These molecules have also been found to stimulate immune function and thus help reduce the pain and inflammation of arthritis. As with glucosamine, it takes time for these nutrients to enter the damaged areas and help to reconstruct the joints. Keep in mind, too, that during the healing process, joints continue to be subjected to activity and stress bearing. Therefore, the benefits of cartilage supplementation tend to be gradual.

There are also some other interesting developments concerning hydrolyzed cartilage. During the last few years there has been a great deal of research into the possibility of the human body's being able to use hydrolyzed cartilage directly after digestion to form new human cartilage tissue.

Much of this research is contradictory owing to some less than exemplary study techniques employed by some of the researchers but it does seem that some of the evidence would lead one to believe that under certain conditions, the human body can use common hydrolyzed cartilage to reform damaged joint tissue.

Methylsulfonylmethane (MSM)

Methylsulfonylmethane (MSM) has been researched since the late 1950's and available as capsules in the healthfood industry for many years. Originally MSM was isolated from various plant (vegetable) sources and discovered to be mildly antiviral in some *in vitro* studies. Further animal studies seemed to show some *in vivo* antiviral effects but expanded human studies proved to be disappointing but some companies continue to sell MSM for this purpose. It is a metabolite of DMSO, and provides all the good effects of DMSO without the drawbacks like the odor on the breath, and drying of the skin when topically applied. MSM has been used historically to treat a wide variety of conditions including allergies, emphysema, arthritis, and some vascular conditions. I use it anywhere that I want to reduce inflammation and enhance circulation.

You may have recently come into contact with methylsulfonylmethane offered as 500 mg. hard-gel capsules in bottles of 180 capsules. Many companies, primarily multilevel, are now offering MSM in this form for various supplementation purposes.

Some Considerations When Purchasing Cetyl Myristoleate (CM)

When trying to determine the quality of this product, there are several considerations. First, the efficacy of the product should be investigated. How long has the product been used? How many people have used the product? What kind of success rates have been noted? Second, what raw material is used for the manufacturing and what is the availability of this material. And third, the total active ingredient (cetyl myristoleate) should be researched. And last, of course, how much does it cost and what other products, if any, are included.

Presently, I know of three manufacturers of cetyl myristoleate. One of the manufacturers uses bovine marrow (fat) as the raw material to obtain its cetyl myristoleate and provides approximately 7.5 grams of active ingredient per treatment. It's marketed in 75 mg. capsules and sells for $295.00 for 100 capsules. The price per gram is $39.34. It is sold without any other joint-restructuring nutrients.

The second manufacturer sells their product in 760 mg. capsules and dosage is recommended according to weight. Under 125 lb. body weight, the recommended treatment is approximately 10 capsules and ends up costing $27.96 per gram.

For larger individuals, they recommend up to 24 capsules which would cost over $500.00. They also use an animal source for their raw material, and there is no adjunctive nutrition supplied or recommended.

The third manufacturer sells their cetyl myristoleate products in various forms, including liquid, and hard & soft gel capsules. They are packaged with two other products, including one which helps rebuild damaged joint cartilage, containing glucosamine, hydrolyzed cartilage, sea cucumber extract, and methylsulfonylmethane (MSM); and a topical cream containing cetly myristoleate to be applied over involved areas of pain. The entire three product package retails for around $150.00. The primary product contains a one-month supply of 18 grams of cetyl myristoleate in liquid gel capsules and 72 grams of other mixed fatty acid esters, of which 60% have synergistic antiarthritic activity. Assuming the other two products (support capsules and lotion) add $50.00 to the total cost of the package, the cost of the 18 grams of cetyl myristoleate is $5.55 per gram.

In addition, unlike the other two more expensive products that I have investigated, this manufacturer uses no toxic acids and solvents such as benzene and acetone to manufacture its product. And this company uses vegetable oil starting material.

Complementary Treatment And Prevention Of Arthritis

There are many other factors to consider when treating and trying to prevent arthritic symptoms from returning. The primary considerations would be diet and nutrition (including possible food allergies), elimination of poisons or toxins in the body (referred to as detoxification), proper exercise, and stress reduction.

Diet and Nutrition

I'm going to sound a little bit like your own doctor here: If you're overweight, the nicest thing you can do for those weight-bearing joints is to lose some weight. And as you already know, fad diets don't offer any permanent answers. In fact, some of them have proved and some may yet prove to be very dangerous. The average American is now 4 lbs. heavier since starting all these low-fat diets, which I'm afraid has sent all of us scurrying around for fat substitutes so we can continue to eat our chips, dips, hamburgers, and low-fat cookies. Now is the time to start. As the sports shoe commercial says, "Just Do It!"

There's lots of great information on proper diet, and much of it is now being recommended by the American Heart Association and the American Cancer Society, so I'm not going to elaborate here. However, there are some key factors that I'd like to address. Eat more fruits and vegetables! If available, choose organically grown; they're more likely to contain all the vitamins and minerals needed for healthy tissue growth and contain none of the dangerous pesticides and insecticides that do liver damage.

Eat more cold water fish such as Salmon, Herring (not kippered or pickled), fresh Sardines, Albacore Tuna, and Mackerel. These fish provide sources for omega-3 fatty acids, which decrease the inflammation and pain of arthritis. They also decrease the amount of cholesterol that the liver produces, thus thinning the blood, making clots less likely to form and reducing plaques on the blood vessel walls.

Decrease your meat consumption. Animal meats, especially organ meats, are high in purines which break down into uric acid, the primary cause of gout. Meat is also loaded with the essential fatty acid, arachadonic acid, which actually increases joint inflammation. Of course, meat also contains all the unhealthy fats that lead to obesity, heart disease, some cancers, and it increases inflammatory processes.

Consider being tested for food allergies. Certain plants belonging to the Solanaceae, or nightshade, family are known to increase the symptoms of certain arthritic conditions. The nightshade family includes tomatoes, white potatoes, hot and sweet peppers, eggplant and tobacco. These plants are known to produce crippling conditions in grazing animals. Dairy products, margarine, shortening, caffeine, alcohols, and sugar should also be dramatically reduced or eliminated from your diet.

One of the most important things that you can do to decrease arthritic symptoms and increase your overall well-being is to increase your daily water consumption. Drinking 2 to 3 quarts of distilled water each day will do more for your health than any of my other suggestions. Distilled water is a powerful therapeutic agent. Because of water's ability to attach to other molecules, distilled water, which has nothing attached to the water molecule, can help leach many of the undesired mineral deposits found in your joints and other tissues and organs and help to eliminate them from your body. Be careful with mineral water which provides minerals in a form that your body has difficulty breaking down and using. These minerals then get deposited in your joints, kidneys, and blood vessels. Your body finds it easier to break down minerals that come from fruits and vegetables than minerals that come directly from the ground.

Chronic pains in the body are often indicators of dehydration. Many times we misinterpret our cravings for water and eat more food rather than drinking the water that our body so desperately needs to carry on all of its functions. The next time you find yourself craving something, try drinking a couple of glasses of distilled water. I promise you, it will change your life! A first thought you should have when any pain arises is "my body is severely short of water!"

Detoxification

Your body eliminates toxins through several pathways. There are two forms of toxins, internal and external. Internal toxins are waste products produced by normal metabolic processes in your body. External toxins are poisons that are found in our environment. The FDA has approved over 70,000 chemicals to be used in our environment that are now found in our food, air, and water supplies. Twenty-five per cent of these chemicals are known carcinogens. As we age, the body's abilities to eliminate these poisons is diminished. Organs of elimination include the colon, liver, kidneys, skin and lungs.

Colon

It is critical that we improve the digestion of our food and decrease the delivery of undigested foods to the colon. Remember, one of the causes of rheumatoid arthritis may be due to large molecules of food in unusable forms entering the blood stream and causing a hyper-immune response. Enzyme therapy will be beneficial here. Go to the health food store and buy a formula that includes all of the digestive plant enzymes, including protease, lipase, amylase, and cellulase. The pancreatic enzymes, including trypsin, should also be included. The enzymes should be taken with meals and for those of you with digestive problems, the lipase may be helpful in digesting cetyl myristoleate which is an oil. Also, increasing dietary fiber (fruits and vegetables, again) decreases the time food spends in the digestive tract and is necessary for any beneficial detoxification program. For those of you who do not respond to the shotgun approach of enzyme therapy, please contact your chiropractor or naturopath who specializes in this field. It is a science unto itself.

Liver

Remember your poor old liver is having to work overtime breaking down all those environmental toxins that we encounter every day. So give it a break and reduce your intake of unhealthy fats, refined sugars, and processed foods, especially those with questionable additives, preservatives and colorings. Alcohol and certain drugs, too, cause liver damage. For those of you with a history of alcohol, drug, or steroid use, you may find emulsifying the cetyl myristoleate very difficult, and therefore, it may not have the desired results. If this is the case, supplement the recommended treatment with some bile salts or lecithin, a very effective emulsifier. Just a note—before fats or oils can be broken down and absorbed, they must be emulsified. This is accomplished by the secretion of bile which is manufactured by the liver and stored in the gall bladder. And for those with liver dysfunction, I recommend a combination of milk thistle extract (silymarin), crude licorice extract (glycyrrhizins) astragalus, and schizandra for mild and effective detoxification.

Kidneys

Reducing your salt and meat consumption will help to reduce the stress to the kidneys and keep them functioning at an optimum level during detoxification. Again, reducing your intake of drugs, food additives, and questionable chemicals is essential in helping to remove metabolic waste products and environmental poisons. Your kidneys will really appreciate, also, that 2 to 3 quarts of distilled water you are now drinking.

Skin

Regular hot showers and baths that open the skin's pores while using an abrasive like the loofah sponge will support the skin's efforts in detoxifying. Hot baths with Epsom salts help to draw the toxins out of the body through the skin. And regular exercise to the point of sweating will be very helpful.

Lungs

Part of your regular exercise should include aerobic exercise. I do not agree with the adage "No pain, no gain," especially when trying to improve joint function. All exercise should be performed within the limits of pain. If your exercise starts to become painful, please stop the one that you're doing and go on to your next exercise. You can always put the painful one back into your routine later on. You may, of course, experience some achiness or stiffness after starting any new exercise routine. This is to be expected since you're using some muscles that probably have not been used in some time. Achiness is all right, pain is not! Swimming and isometric exercises are probably the most effective without doing further damage to your joints.

Another exercise that is extremely powerful and—like switching to distilled water—will change your life is performing deep-breathing exercises. Deep breathing will provide oxygen to parts of your lungs that have not experienced fresh air in ages. It will also stimulate fresh blood supply to the now newly reactivated parts of your lungs and increase the body's abilities to rid itself of volatile substances. Of course, aerobic exercise like swimming and jogging can do all of the above, but not to the degree like the focused breathing exercise that I'll describe below. I'm not an advocate of jogging since it can cause further damage to all your weight-bearing joints.

If you must jog, please wear the proper shoes to absorb shock and keep the proper biomechanics of your feet; custom orthotics that fit inside your shoes can be helpful here. Run on earth or sand surfaces, not on pavement or asphalt, and pick a location to run where you will not be forced to breathe automobile or factory exhausts. The Good Lord gave us only one liver to handle all these toxins!

My favorite breathing exercise is simple, but powerful. Try and do this three times a day. If you can't do it three times, do it twice or even once. But do it! Find a quiet place where you won't be interrupted for five minutes. You can even do this in your car, but please shut off your ignition, of course, before you walk into you work place. This might even make going to work a little easier! Take a deep breath through your nose filling both your upper lung lobes and the lower lobes. You must use your diaphragm to do this so your stomach must protrude outwards and your chest must expand on full inhalation. Now hold it in for a count of four. Release your breath slowly through your mouth for twice as long as you inhaled. This will ensure that all of the air with the toxins, like carbon dioxide, get out of your system. In other words, if you inhale to a count of eight, hold for a count of four, and exhale for a count of sixteen. The numbers are arbitrary. Do what feels comfortable. Repeat this process ten times and, like I said, try to do it three times a day. If you do this for one month, I guarantee you will no longer have the same body.

Some Final Thoughts

The one factor that seems to be the most important during the healing process of any physical ailment is attitude. I'm always hesitant to use numbers in describing anything so subjective as health, but if I were to try and objectify attitude, it would be, at least, 70% of the healing process. I have seen patients overcome insurmountable odds by becoming actively involved in their own care and heal from so-called incurable diseases. On the flip side, I have had patients who have stinkin' thinkin' and never recover from minor ailments that should have been resolved years ago.

Attitude not only means trying to hold a good thought during the healing, it means taking control of your own body, maybe for the first time in your life, and becoming an active participant. Educate yourselves by asking your doctor questions, go to the library, or search the Internet on your computer. The information you gather will empower you to take an active role in your healing and remaining well. Look at disease not as something bad that has happened to you, but as an opportunity to dig a little deeper into yourself to find those inner strengths and the source of healing.

Please do not expect your physician to heal you; healing comes from within. If you have a great doctor, he or she may know what buttons to push to remove the obstacles to healing and maybe even teach you how to prevent future disease, but you must furnish that healing power.

Good luck and God speed on your road to recovery! By the way, I always thought that God traveled at the speed of light, but when it comes to healing, sometimes He travels a little slower. Be patient, travel slower yourself, be with yourself, and you may find that you really enjoy your own company!

FREQUENTLY ASKED QUESTIONS

What is cetyl myristoleate?

Cetyl myristoleate is the common name for *cis-9*-cetyl myristoleate. It is a completely natural substance found in certain animals, including beavers and mice. As supplied, it is a naturally derived, highly purified, and refined waxy ester prepared for oral administration.

How does cetyl myristoleate work?

Some authors and practitioners believe that cetyl myristoleate has the ability to reprogram faulty memory T-cells, thus treating the cause of arthritis. I have not found this to be totally correct. Cetyl myristoleate seems to have the ability to normalize hyper-immune responses, thus the favorable results in treating autoimmune conditions such as rheumatoid arthritis and systemic lupus erythematosus, but it seems to function more effectively as a surfactant, or lubricant, and a powerful anti-inflationary. My recommended protocol also provides natural synergistic nutrients that start immediately to help reconstruct damaged joint tissue. Although the major benefits come promptly, minor improvements continue for several months after finishing the one-month long program.

Is it harmful in any way?

Cetyl myristoleate studies began at the U.S. National Institutes for Health more than 25 years ago. Recently, clinical application studies were conducted by the San Diego Clinic. No harmful short- or long-term effects were ever observed in humans or in laboratory animals, even in extremely high doses. Similar substances have been used in common foods, including cheese and chocolate and even in medicines and cosmetics. It is a perfectly safe, naturally derived substance.

Does the protocol work for both rheumatoid and osteoarthritis?

Both types of arthritis respond equally well. The program that I suggest, which includes the mixed fatty acid esters (including cetyl myristoleate), joint support capsules, and topical cream has also been found effective in treating other forms of arthritic conditions including gout, ankylosing spondylitis, Reiter's syndrome, Sjogren's syndrome, and psoriasis. It has also been found to relieve various types of back pain of undetermined origin, which is more than likely arthritis-related.

Does your recommended protocol improve joint mobility?

Absolutely! If the joint can be moved just slightly, by either the afflicted person or even by someone else, joint mobility can usually be restored. However, if the bones have fused, only surgery may restore joint function.

Does the recommended protocol stop arthritis pain?
Arthritis pain will disappear if the total protocol is followed. In a few extreme cases, pain can be reduced by only 70% to 90%. This generally, however, provides sufficient benefit to allow the person to function normally again.

How long is it before benefits are noticed?
Most people begin to feel relief within ten to fourteen days. Others may take a bit longer and a few may even need six to eight weeks.

Can it correct deformities?
Yes. Deformed fingers and toes are often caused by inflammation which swells joints and pushes the bones out of place. Reduction of the swelling improves appearance dramatically and often allows the subluxated bones to return to their normal position. Extreme cases may require some physical therapy.

What about really severe cases?
Severe cases may require a follow-up treatment. I suggest waiting several weeks after completing a one-month course of cetyl myristoleate while continuing the other support capsules (glucosamine, etc.). Some people may find they need to take a few capsules now and then to retain their improvement. After treatment is completed, most severe cases, including those confined to bed and wheelchairs, find that they no longer have to depend on others for their care.

Does it work for everyone?
So far, the treatment that I recommend has been effective in treating all arthritic conditions unless the user has had a history of liver dysfunction. Liver impairment can be caused by diseases, such as hepatitis, alcohol or drug abuse. In these cases, bile salts or lecithin may be helpful in emulsifying the cetyl myristoleate. And the enzyme lipase may help in breaking down the oil so that it can be absorbed.

Can I continue with my usual medications?
Yes, but after a few days, you may find that you won't need them. However, it's best to avoid steroids if possible. You can check with your doctor.

Is age a factor?
Not really. All ages respond well. Although arthritis is far more common in adults, even young children are sometimes afflicted. With small children start with one half of the recommended dose and increase slowly to a regular dose.

References:

"Antiinflammatory Diet in Rheumatic Disease". Adam, O. *European Journal of Clinical Nutrition*, 1995.

"Botanical Lipids". *Effects in Inflammation, Immune Response, and Rheumatoid Arthritis".* Rothman. D., et al. Seminars in Arthritis and Rheumatism, October 1995.

"Cetyl Myristoleate Isolated from Swiss Albino Mice: An Apparent Protective Agent against Adjuvant Arthritis in Rats". Diehl, H., and May, E.L. *Journal of Pharmaceutical Science, Vol. 83,* March 1994.

"Effects of High Dose Fish Oil on Rheumatoid Arthritis after Stopping Nonsteroidal Antiinflammatory Drugs". Kremer, J., MD, *Arthritis and Rheumatism,* August 1995.

"Effects of Modulation of Inflammatory and Immune Parameters in Patients with Rheumatic and Inflammatory Disease Receiving Dietary Supplementation of N-3 and N-6 Fatty Acids". Kremer, J., MD, *Lipids*, 1996.

"Glycosaminoglycan Supplements as Therapeutic Agents". Bucci, L., PhD., *Nutritional Report*, January 1996.

"Rheumatoid Arthritis and Foods: A Patient Study"., Borok, G., *South African Family Practice*, October 1989.

"The Biological Activity of Bovine Cartilage Preparations". Prudden, J. MD, Balassa, L., *Seminars in Arthritis and Rheumatism*, Summer 1974.

" U.S. Patent *#4049824*, September 20, 1977, Cetyl Myristoleate.